Principles of Healthy Menu Development

Katherine A. A. Zupan

Flying Finish Press

ISBN 978-0-359-92414-1

ISBN 978-0-359-92414-1 90000

9 780359 924141

"If you understand the science, figuring out what to eat is easy."

- Dr. Jason Fung

Introduction

Telling the tale of losing weight & preserving health.

Chapter One
From "gluttony & sloth" to "zealotry & greed".
French Paradox, Club Med & Eating Nordic

Chapter Two
Establishing menu goals
Bioavailability

Chapter Three
The importance of diversity & sustain-ability
Macronutrients' culinary roles
Micronutrients' culinary roles

Chapter Four
The Optimal Human Diet
The New Food Pyramid

Introduction

The optimal way of feeding humans has been the subject of greatest scientific and popular interest for the past century. The debates are not quite over yet, but the evidence clearly indicates that most of the world's current diets are not optimal as indicated by rising levels of heart disease, diabetes and obesity worldwide.

The USDA dietary guidelines, promoting 50% of daily calories coming from carbohydrates, are not correct and weren't from inception but, until now, the science of human biochemistry hasn't been able to speak with knowledge and authority on the subject. Now it can. Humans need to eat nutrient dense natural foods, restrict carbohydrates, and avoid industrially processed, man-made foods to be heathy. Despite lingering controversy, one thing remains clear.

You cannot outrun a poor diet.

Chapter One

Look at the evidence. Despite 50 years spent demonizing fat while pushing statins and stents, heart disease remains the number one killer worldwide. Diabetes is close behind. The costs of caring for these metabolic diseases, and the loss of productivity, is bankrupting nations to the point where banks and the military are taking notice and complaining. Lifespans are shortening. Still, doctors promoting and recommending ketogenic diets are being prosecuted because they are having an impact upon major food manufacturers' profits and threatening their government subsidies that enable them to cheaply grow and sell to us the food that is killing us. The greed of corporations is astounding.

Until the guidelines change, nothing will be done. The latest panel assembled to review the guidelines explains why nothing will be done. Representatives of the corporations, doctors supported by corporations, lobbyists paid by corporations and Seventh Day Adventists who have joined with Animal Rights activists and vegans form the bulk of the committee and the witness/consultant list. The current committee has also declined to add the latest biochemical and medical research to their evidence list. Hopes for real guideline change grow dim. Zealotry and greed will prevail and human shamed for their gluttony and sloth. "It is your fault you're fat."

No, it isn't. The advice we were given was and still is wrong.

There has been some change for the better. Sugar is now restricted. Still too high, but it's a start. The American Medical Association (AMA) and the American College of Cardiology (ACC) no longer consider cholesterol to be of medical interest and the Obesity Medicine Association (OMA) and the ACC both regard the ketogenic diet, and the Mediterranean diet, to be useful for reducing obesity and heart disease so small yet significant progress has been made. However, the interplay of diet and metabolism has been known for the past 100 years.

The French Paradox invalidated Dr. Ansel Keys' hypothesis that dietary fat caused heart disease. The French eat a great deal more fat but have less heart disease. Further, this paradox is one of many.

Currently, the healthiest diet (way of eating) is thought to be the Mediterranean Diet especially when coupled to a 'dulce vita' laid-back lifestyle. A few years ago, we were told to eat as the Icelanders did by increasing the amount of fish in our diet. The Fukushima Daiichi nuclear power plant meltdown put an end to that.

The latest efforts on the meatless front include Asia and the creation of laboratory-made 'fake meat' that includes heme. Oh good, synthetic meat...not. Asia's medical training is being changed to comply with the dietary rules of the Seventh Day Adventists which were created by a woman in the 1860's to stop the heinous sin of masturbation which in her unscientific mind led to weakness, insanity and early death. The company Sanctuary is a wholly-owned subsidiary of the church and therefore is a 'for profit but tax-free' company. Sanctuary is running the medical education effort in Asia.

Will we soon be told to eat fake meat out of the vat and monocropped plants that ruin the fertility of the soil because of religious dogma and animal rights zeal or will real not 'corporate' science prevail?

Chapter Two

With the history out of the way, we can now concentrate upon how the individual can go about building a healthy menu.

First, establish your goals. Do this by focusing upon who you're feeding and their health. What do they really need to eat that they will in fact eat and what in particular must they avoid eating?

Nutritional ketogenic diets stress eating animal-based saturated fats, meats, fish, berries and nuts, full-fat dairy, vegetables that grow above the ground, and leafy green salads with vinaigrette dressings made using olive oil.

The Mediterranean diet includes all of the above, but focusing more on fish than meat, along with wine, pasta, fruit (not juice) and various baked goods.

Many people switch between the two, using ketogenic diets to restore their health and lose weight and then 'going Med' for maintenance. An importance difference between the two is ketogenic diets decrease the amount of protein, regardless of source, limiting consumption to 1 gram per kilo of lean body mass per day.

If you do prefer a more plant-based diet, you will require supplementation of B12 and choline to stay healthy. Yes, vegans can do keto but doing that requires more work.

Step two is making notes of what you have learned then seeing what is locally available that you can afford. Grass-fed, pasture-raised, wild-caught, free-range and certified organic foods are best, but they cost more. Buy the best you can afford. You don't have to eat premium quality to get the results. It will simply take a bit longer to get there. Stay within your budget.

Next, clean out your kitchen by removing all the banned foods, including those that are doubtful. Also remove all so-called 'vegetable oils', implicated in dementia and Alzheimer's, and soy products, which are endocrine disruptors. Beware condiments. And get rid of fruit juices. Whole fruit is better for you and home-grown and heritage is best. Grow your vegetables if you can.

Remove all processed foods such as Kraft macaroni and cheese. No fake foods. If it comes in a box chances are you shouldn't be eating it because when they took the fat out, they put sugar in to make it taste good. Remember fat carries the flavor of the food.

Then, bring in all the foods you and yours will now be eating. But you may be wondering what those healthy saturated fats might be.

Healthy Saturated Fats:

Lard (pork)   Suet (sheep/goats)
Tallow (cows)   Butter (dairy)

Coconut oil and olive oil are the plant-based options. Omega-3 fats are gotten by eating fish or the best cod liver oil in capsules which is taken as a supplement.

Avocados and palm kernel oils are also permitted but I cannot recommend them because they are not being sustainably grown and are wreaking havoc upon the environments.

Applying this to meat, especially ruminants, I follow Allan Savory's protocol which improves the soil and stops desertification caused by monocropping and thus, is sustainable.

Why is a vegan ketogenic diet laborious? Because the nutrients in the plants are less bioavailable to humans and plants contain phytotoxins that can harm the gut. This means you have to eat more plants to get fed while increasing the risk of destroying your intestinal wall thus creating 'leaky gut' which allows the gut biome, both the good and the bad, to enter your bloodstream where they do not belong. You cannot simply assume that you aren't sensitive to certain phytotoxins and you cannot assume that repeated use in the amounts required will not cause an increase in your sensitivity to them over time. I understand you have your reasons, but it is not a wise choice.

Bioavailability

Raw navy beans contain more protein than raw beef does, per 100 grams. However, raw beans are toxic to humans. Once properly cooked, the beef contains more protein than the beans. Why?

Because the protein in the beef is more bio-available to humans. This is why most plant foods have to be eaten in larger quantities to get what you need and, if processed, must be fortified with synthetic nutrients. Read the label and yes, fortification is required by law.

Be advised that plants can only contain the nutrients they get from the soil in which they are grown, hence the need for fertilizers most of which come from petroleum. Washing in clean water is recommended. Trimming may also be required, for example rhubarb. Rhubarb is a tasty vegetable, usually used like a fruit, but the leaves are toxic. Cashews, delicious as they are, in their hulls are outright poisonous and have to hulled by machine. You can buy walnuts in their hulls, but you cannot find unhulled cashews for this reason.

Plants develop these phytotoxins because they really do not want to be eaten and they cannot run away from those who want to eat them. Hence, pesticides, most of which also come from petrol-eum. We risk phytotoxins to get phytonutrients.

Humans long ago traded in big guts for a big brain, nature having decreed one or the other but not both because each is metabolically expensive. This trade-off requires humans to each nutrient dense foods like meat and saturated fats both of which give us more 'bang for a buck' per gram aka foods of greater bioavailability. Greater bio-availability means you can eat smaller amounts of these foods, making it easier and less costly to get all the nutrients you need.

However there are a few caveats you cannot ignore when it comes to animal-based diets. You have to limit the amount of wild rabbit and polar bear liver that you eat, and meat must be fresh or properly preserved. The animal must also be healthy and without parasites. The devout religious also may have prohibitions about certain meats. Such as the injunction for Catholics to eat only fish on Fridays which is why MacDonald's developed and still sell their Filet o' Fish sand-wich. The fish they use changes with availability and that depends upon what fish is in season and how much fishermen are permitted to harvest.

In most of the developed nations, we suffer from abundance despite also having food deserts in which our marginalized and poor citizens live. We have to do better to make healthy, bio-available foods more widely available.

Chapter Three

We've touched on the topics earlier, but now it is time to get serious and in depth about how the foods we eat are grown, prepared for sale and marketed. We have to decide which it is we want farming real food on fertile lands or food manufactured in factories and laboratories. Due to past experiences, all food intended for public consumption in the US is regulated.

In the US, all meat, regardless of species, is inspected and graded by the USDA to various extents as required by law. This also includes the farms, the feeds, and the butchering facilities as well. All beef cattle are raised on grass with supplements as needed. Then they are all grain-finished in feedlots for their final 3 to 6 months of life. Nowadays, people hate killing animals for food. Dairy and egg production are not exempt from regulation. The problem with dairy and egg production is 'the useless male'. We eat male cattle, but we mostly make pet food from the male chicks instead of raising capons. Male turkeys are travesties of genetic engineering, all breast and drumsticks.

Contrary to popular opinion, nothing is wasted. Scraps become various processed meats or pet food. This too is regulated. Then there are pigs who will eat anything. The only waste occurs in the home.

Most meat species are raised on less fertile soil on rangelands and grasslands that are not suitable for crops. The fertility can be improved over time by pasturing and moving cattle in a more tightly herded way, but this requires manpower, careful planning and monitoring. It also takes time.

All plants are raised as large acreage monocrops because this makes it easier to use machinery. Irrigation, pesticides, herbicides and fungicides may be required. Bees are intensively used as pollinators, at risk of their lives, from the various poisons, see above, routinely 'dusted' on these crops. Honey from these bees is discarded. Small creatures are inadvertently killed during harvest.

All farming is 'at risk' from the weather. But commodity prices and fluctuations in the market increase this risk making farming an 'always on the edge of bankruptcy' business despite crop insurance. Enter government subsidies because people gotta eat. It doesn't do the politicians any good if famine kills off their voters on their watch. All of the above has led us to where we are today. Fortunes can be made, and bankruptcy can be staved off to next year but there's no denying that the way food is grown in America is unsustainable and the farmland's growing less fertile.

Soil needs a diverse biome to be fertile. This biome needs to fed organic matter, protected from erosion by wind, it needs water that doesn't run off and it needs to rest, beneath a nitrogen-fixing cover crop, until the biome has recovered. Crop seeds must be drilled in leaving the soil untilled. Dusting with various petroleum-based poisons is not desirable. Compaction of the soil by the weight of heavy machinery is not desirable but animal-drawn equipment is too slow, easily ex-hausted and requires greater care and too few people know how to work a team.

I wish to ignore politics, but this isn't possible because we have to consider taxation but to keep it as simple as possible, both income and the land that enables making the income are annually taxed. Operating expenses, machinery depre-ciation can all help reduce the tax, but taxes rarely go and stay away.

Then there is the question of subsidies. Why are grains and sugar production subsidized? Because for decades poor people, mainly in the south, were slowly dying due to poor nutrition and the diseases thereof. The easiest thing to was to fortify the grains. A 'let them eat bread' solution because that's pretty much all they could afford to buy. Wheat, corn, oats, rye and barley were subsidized to induce manufacturers to increase production. Kellogg, a Seventh Day Adventist, was ecstatic.

The biochemical science of nutrition was poorly understood. European scientists were investigating the impact of hormones upon the body's nutritional requirements while the Americans and some others were busy thinking about the 2nd Law of Thermodynamics and nutrition versus exercise. But after World War II, all European science had been discredited by the Nazi's.

Then grains and sugar won the fight for the money by using Ansel Keys' hypothesis that saturated fat gave us heart disease and the alliance between the Seventh Day Adventists, animal rights activists, vegetarians and vegans emotional -based beliefs. Proctor and Gamble had already ousted lard with their ads for made from cottonseeds Crisco, so the public was primed and ready to believe almost anything was more 'modern' and 'healthy' than the 'old-fashioned' stuff their grandmothers and great grandmothers had used. Now it was meat, dairy, egg and tropical oil producers that would be denigrated.

Grains are still king, soybeans have gained, and sugar has seen its position eroded since then 1980's. But we are still stuck with Ansel Keys' not merely unproven but discredited hypothesis and the nutritional guidelines based upon it because the emotional-based beliefs remain. No one wants to remember that life on earth is cyclical because that means death is required for life and plants' lives are more easily taken.

But the soil can't endure feeding monocrops forever. Desertification is a growing problem even in the American Midwest. Reliance upon grains is also having a detrimental impact upon human health because plants contain less nutrition than humans need unless eaten in bulk and in combination. This requires more plants to be grown on more and increasingly less fertile land. All of this makes American agriculture less diverse and less sustainable. Subsidies must be changed to support the nutritional foods human really do need to meet their needs. These are mainly animal-based foods as a now matured, biochemical-based nutritional science shows. We still need vegetables, but we do not need to eat at least half of our daily calories from complex carbohydrates and 100 pounds of sugar per person per year as we now do. The unsustainability of current agriculture is reflected in the unsustainability of the nutritional guide-lines and the unsustainability of the standard American diet.

How is this to be done in the home?
Decrease the use of grains, tubers and sugar.
Increase the use of vegetables grown above the ground and buy organic sustainably raised if you

can afford to do so or grow your own vegetables if you can.

Buy foods locally produced on farms, not factories. Support farms, not factories.

The Macronutrients

Macronutrients provide most of our energy and nutrition. The three are meat, fat and carbohydrates. Meat and fat are nutritionally dense, essential on a daily basis and the nutrition they supply is highly bioavailable. Carbohydrates are not nutritionally dense, as sold, unless fortified, are not essential for most humans and the nutrition they supply is less bioavailable.

Currently, most people use carbohydrates for energy production but there are those who require some carbohydrates to sustain their lives, the type 1 diabetics. The rest of us can make all the carbohydrates we need which is why carbohydrates are not essential. The human liver breaks down fat to make carbohydrates as needed to fuel the cells that do not have mitochondria such as red blood cells. Carbohydrates and meat, when used for energy, give us 4 kilocalories per gram. Fat used for energy gives us 9 kcal/gram, more than twice as much yet we senselessly cut if off our meat because we think it is bad for us despite all evidence to the contrary.

Meat provides the essential amino acids we need to live. Various fats provide the essential fatty acids we need to live. Were you aware that the fat in beef and pork is half saturated and half monounsaturated? Thinking about polyunsaturated oils, did you know there are two varieties, omega-3 and omega-6, and that you need both of them? Fat is complicated but if you do not eat meat and fatty fish, you're not getting all of the fats you need to be healthy. The proteins in meat and fish are mainly used to build and repair your body while the fat content supports cholesterol production.

Cholesterol we can make on our own as we do with carbohydrates. Our bodies only make what is needed. If more is eaten, the body's production is decreased, if less then production is increased to meet requirements. Eating more merely means less work for your body. Cholesterol used to build and repair cell walls, amongst other things including transportation of nutrients and energy in the bloodstream. Only animal-based foods give us cholesterol, a type of fat. The AMA is no longer concerned about cholesterol as of 2018.

Culinary uses of the macronutrients.

Carbohydrates: grains, vegetables. fruits and sugars.

Grains provide bulk, energy, thickening, fiber and structure.

Vegetables provide phytonutrients, bulk, phyto-toxins and fiber.

Fruits provide phytonutrients, sweetness and fiber

Sugars provide sweetness, caramelization, self-life, energy and structure.

Fiber is said to be good for us because it feeds the gut thus aiding in proper elimination. Constipation is blamed on a lack of fiber in the diet. Yes, and no, but truth be told, fiber's only value is the time it takes to move through the gut and that can become a bad thing with too much being worse than too little. We don't need as much as we typically eat, and you can do without any. The mucus produced by the gut is a response to damage to the gut by fiber. The intestinal wall is meant to protect us from the microbes in our gut. Too much damage leads to leaky gut which lets these biome get into the bloodstream and this can kill. So be careful about how much fiber you include in your menu.

All carbohydrates become sugar in the body.

Grains = glucose   Tubers = dextrose
Fruits = fructose   Sugars = sucrose

Corn contains starch, dextrose, so it is considered a tuber – a starchy vegetable – although it is modified grain. Corn, in any form, is not permit-ted in any quantity.

Onions, which grow below the ground, contain sugar, sucrose, yet they are permitted in small quantities to enhance the flavor of other foods. They also contain vitamin C.

Legumes, regardless of how they are grown are mostly starch, dextrose, and despite their protein content, are not permitted in any form or quantity. This group includes most peas and most beans. Green beans are excepted. Green peas are not, as odd as that seems. Biochemistry is complicated.

Berries and citrus fruits are permitted in very limited quantities on an occasional basis. These fruits contain lower levels of sugar with higher than average fiber and massive amounts of vitamin C. They are also highly antiangiogenic, hence their inclusion. All other fruits are exclude-ed.

Be advised that through centuries of selective breeding, all grains, fruits and vegetables are modified versions of their original forms. Humans made them into what they are now and genetic modification by humans will continue to make them into what we want them to be. Which is to say that the word 'natural' will become increasingly meaningless.

<u>Meats</u>: animals, fishes and birds, nuts and eggs.

Animals and birds provide amino acids, gristle, bone and marrow, various fatty acids, vitamins especially B12 and choline. Birds and lizards also provide eggs.

Fishes provide omega-3 fatty acids, eggs, amino acids and vitamins.

Eggs are considered to be perfect foods because they contain everything one needs in a highly bioavailable form in one easily handled, package.

Nuts are seeds encased in hulls. (Fruits are seeds encased in flesh.) They contain vary amounts of all three macronutrients but are most valued for their protein and fat content. Peanuts are legumes, not nuts. Fatty nuts in small quantities are allowed.

Insects are eaten by some people, but they do have a high "ick" factor which renders their nutrient content immaterial. Promoters for their inclusion in our diets do exist. However, part of developing a healthy diet is considering what people want to eat and if a strong negative visceral reaction is received, it is best to not include that item on one's menu.

Bones, bone marrow, gristle and offal aka organ meats are all important sources of nutrition that require more than the usual amount of proper handling. Bones are first roasted, have their meat and marrow removed, and then are slowly stewed for their gelatin and mineral content. Gristle needs chewing but it helps keep the ligaments holding one's joints together healthy. Organ meats are rich in nutrients sometimes to the point of excess. Polar bear liver is so rich in Vitamin A that it is toxic to humans. Various organs contain varying amounts of each nutrient, but they all contain many of them. Yes, there are those who will refuse to eat them. One can but try.

Amino acids are organic compounds mainly composed of carbon, hydrogen, oxygen and nitrogen. There are 500 amino acids known that occur naturally. As proteins, they are the largest component in the human body and also play a significant roles in various processes such as in neurotransmitter transportation and biosynthesis.

Nine proteinogenic amino acids are called "essential" for humans because they cannot be produced from other compounds by the human body and so must be taken in as food, these are phenylalanine, valine, threonine, tryptophan, methionine, leucine, isoleucine, lysine, and histidine. Despite current opinions, animal-based sources are inherently more complete and more bioavailable than plant-based sources. Meat gives substance to a meal.

Fats: saturated, monounsaturated, polyunsaturated omega-3 and polyunsaturated omega-6.

Saturated fats have all or predominantly single bonds. They are solid at room temperature and have higher melting points. They are slow to oxidize (go rancid). There are approximately 45 saturated fats. Cholesterol is made from saturated fats. Stable at higher (cooking) temperatures.

Monounsaturated fats (MUFAs) have one double bond, are fast to oxidize and liquid at room temperature. There are 12 monounsaturated fats. Somewhat unstable at higher temperatures.

Polyunsaturated fats (PUFAs) have two or more double bonds, come in *cis-* or *trans-* forms and are omega-3 or omega-6. Highly unstable at higher temperatures and are always liquid. While available in nature, such as in fish and seafood, most are industrially produced from seeds, not vegetables as they are called in advertisements. They require hydrogenation to prevent them from auto-oxidizing. Most are used in industrial applications.

Fatty acids are both important dietary sources of fuel for animals and they are important structural components for cells. When metabolized, by the mitochondria of the cell, fatty acids yield large quantities of ATP. Saturated fats are essential for the formation of cholesterol, also needed for life. The essential fatty acids humans need to support life, are found in many sources: fish and certain seaweeds for omega-3 fats and animals, tropical oils and nuts for omega-6 fats. If this were all, and one considered from an 'essentiality' viewpoint, an entirely carnivorous diet is just as healthy, if not more so, as is a vegan diet. Fats carry the flavor and 'mouth-feel' to a meal but they also trigger satiation. Eating meat without fat leads to a condition called 'protein poisoning' or rabbit starvation, wild rabbit meat having no fat, which leads to 'fat hunger', an irresistible craving for fat, and to death if left untreated.

Humans have been around for 300,000 years and yet agriculture only began in 10,000 BCE. It is foolish to think that the foods we had previously been eating all those years, mostly meats and fats, somehow became 'bad' for us in the late 1950's. There were no farms or orchards during the Ice Ages. Winters, floods, locusts, droughts and other natural occurring problems are not kind to crops. People in many regions still have to eat what they can get. This makes relying upon the most nutrient dense foods the prudent choice, meaning meats with fats should be central in our diet.

Balanced Macronutrient Intake

Fats = 60% of daily caloric requirement
        From natural sources

Protein = 1 gram per kilo of lean body mass
From natural, organic, grass-fed, pasture-raised, wild-caught or gathered sources

Carbohydrate = maximum of 20 grams per day
Limited to non-starchy vegetables, leafy greens, and dairy sources. No processed foods the come in a box or package and nothing low-fat.

Note: limiting the ingestion of carbohydrates released stored water which takes salt with it. Salt intake should be increased to retain required electrolytes.

Culinary Roles of Micronutrients

Providing us with needed vitamins and minerals is the main role of crop vegetables and salad vegetables. Vitamins and minerals have important roles in how well bodily processes run.

In human nutrition iodine, iron, zinc, folate, sodium and vitamin A are of special importance for pregnant women, infants and children.

The most common way to get iodine, sodium, chloride, magnesium and potassium is as salts while vitamin A and heme iron come from meats.

Care must be taken to neither under nor overdo minerals and the fat-soluble vitamins such as vitamin A. Water-soluble vitamins, such as vitamin C, can be under done but any excesses are simply excreted.

Fat-soluble vitamins are A, D, E and K.

Water-soluble vitamins are C and all of the 8 B vitamins. Boiling any foods rich in these vitamins result in deficiency unless the water they are boiled in is included in the meal itself.

However, antinutrients, those compounds that prevent the uptake of needed nutrients by the human body, are disabled by cooking.

Each vitamin has several forms and each of those separate forms may have variants for example vitamin K comes in K1 and K2 both do different things, K1 makes blood coagulation possible, while K2 regulates calcium deposition. K2 comes in many variants, with mk4 and mk7 being the variants humans can use.

Certain minerals require the presence of certain of vitamins to act as buffering agents. Calcium requires vitamin D3 for example.

It can all get very complicated, but the correct balance can be achieved without effort by following the optimum human diet.

Chapter Four

The Optimum Human Diet

The most nutritious diet for the average healthy human being is one that includes the widest variety of natural, nutrient dense foods while strictly limiting the amount of carbohydrates and moderating the amount of proteins ingested.

As a general minimum standard for most people, a 2000 caloric requirement should be met by eating: 60% fat, 20% protein, 10% non-starch vegetables, 5% dairy and 5% nuts and low-glycemic fruits all on a per person per day basis.

1,200 calories worth of healthy fats, mostly-animal-based. Translated into ounces, this equals about 5 ounces per person per day.[1]

400 calories of proteins which is 4 ounces per person per day.[2]

200 calories from vegetables or 50 grams or 2 ounces.

---

[1] 1200kcal divided by 9kcal/gram = 133.33 which equals 4.7 ounces.
[2] 400kcal divided by 4kcal/gram = 100 which equals 3..5 ounces.

100 calories of dairy = or one 10-fl oz glass of whole milk[3]

100 calories of berries or nuts or 1 ounce. But this last 5% can be called "other" because this is where antioxidants, treats, and antiangiogenic foods are placed.

Surprised? It doesn't look like much, but this is the minimum any healthy human needs to survive if they drink enough clean fresh water. This is why most people who eat a nutritional ketogenic diet eat only one meal a day (OMAD), why strict carnivore dieters can remain perfectly healthy and why some vegans can survive as well. You do not really need to eat as much as you do if total carbohydrates are limited to 20 grams per day.

But if one isn't healthy or if one's taking medications for a certain condition or disease, a doctor's supervision becomes mandatory. Even then, however, care must be taken to keep one's reliance upon carbohydrates as low as one can.

---

[3] If lactose tolerant. Dairy is included because it is, like eggs, a whole food – containing fat, protein, minerals and vitamins.

Remember that metabolic diseases/disorders are cause by abundance and the eating of excessive amounts of carbohydrates.

Mixing sugar and fats results in oxidation of the fat in the blood which then builds up and blocks arteries. Since you need fat to live and you don't need the carbohydrates, the wise choice is to drop the carbohydrates thus preventing this oxidation. In short, no sugar = no heart attacks.

Excess protein can induce gluconeogenesis, the transformation of proteins into carbohydrates. So, moderate one's protein intake and stay below the gluconeogenic limit. Less protein = fewer carbo-hydrates = fewer heart attacks.

Yes, the fat content appears to be very high but at 5 ounces, it really isn't. The trick here is a biochemical one. Burning fat doesn't turn into sugar, it turns into ketones instead. Both the brain and the heart prefer being fueled by ketones because they are 'clean' and their use requires less oxygen, leaving more oxygen available for other processes and functions. Carbohydrates are a messy, oxygen-hungry and water-loving fuel. Ketones, specifically beta-hydroxybutyrate, is the body's "dream" fuel or 'more pay for less work". That's the difference between 9kcal/gram in fat and a measly 4 kcal/gram in carbohydrate. Put down the toast, eat the bacon.

Now then, the problems with man-made PUFAs is their involvement with degenerative mental conditions such as Alzheimer's and dementia. This is why only animal sources, ex. oily fishes, are recommended. Unfortunately, we are a long way from a cure but MCT oil taken daily can help hold the degeneration off, but the inevitable will eventually occur.

Diabetes can be reversed, but not cured. The damage to the body caused by diabetes cannot be fixed, so the plan is to prevent the death of one's pancreatic beta cells by giving them time off before one develops full blown diabetes. Insulin highly reacts to carbohydrates, reacts a little to proteins and doesn't care at all about fats. The idea is to 'flat-line' one's insulin by eating zero carbohydrates. No sugar = no insulin = no diabetes and no non-alcoholic fatty liver disease (NAFLD). Excess sugar is stored as fat in organs where it doesn't belong by insulin.

These diseases and conditions are all facets of Metabolic Syndrome which is a new umbrella term for what used to be called "carbohydrate intolerance". Each of these conditions represents a form of metabolic mayhem and they are all the product of eating more carbohydrates than one needs for a long period of time. Exercise and low-fat diets have nothing to do with it and cannot fix any of these diseases. The only diet that will work is one the requires carbohydrate restriction.

You can't outrun a poor diet.

Nutritional Ketogenic Food Pyramid

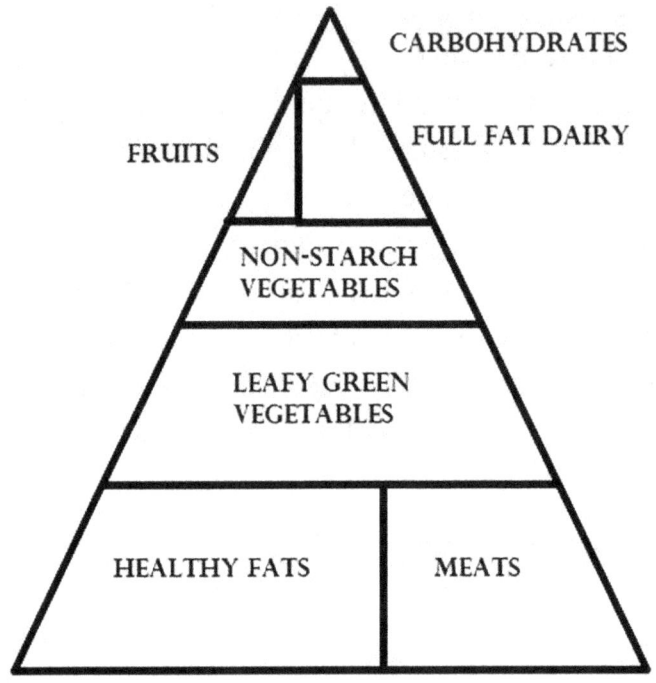

Begin with 60% of daily caloric expenditure coming from healthy fat and 20% coming from meat then, with 20 grams of carbohydrates being the peak, fulfill the remaining calories required using low glycemic, non-starchy, full-fat, un-processed, natural, grass-fed, organic, pasture-raised, wild-caught and no sugar foods.[4] Include antiangiogenics on a monthly basis to start with.

Depending upon the health of those being fed, some of these recommendations might need to be adjusted to give the maximum benefit to the maximum number of people.

For those living in a mixed household, that is half keto and half not, change the fats used and use substitutes for sugar and starch but otherwise cook as normal and simply omit the carbo-hydrates from the keto people's plates.

For one pot meals, casseroles, stews, soups and so on, either cook a keto version in another pot or use cheese, gelatin, eggs or psyllium husks as the binder as appropriate. Use reduction to thicken to the level desired. To add fat, use butter where you can.

---

[4] See Dr. Westman's Page 4 protocol
https://www.dietdoctor.com/se/wp-content/2014/10/no_sugar_no_starch_diet.pdf

Conclusion

For every benefit there's a cost. When it comes to nutritional ketogenic diets the costs are few while the benefits are tremendous. Happiness, we are told, is the absence of physical pain and psychological turmoil, being free of irrational fears, enjoying life itself and having good friends. Since a nutritional ketogenic diet has been shown to improve three of the four criteria for happiness there's no reason not to go keto even if one's doctor is opposed to the experiment. Certainly the three weeks to six month adaptation period can be onerous but isn't good health worth the effort?

I offer my gratitude to the many doctors who have devoted their lives discovering the truly optimal diet for humans: the nutritional ketogenic diet, with special thanks offered to Dr.s Noakes, Phinney, Fetke and Volek.

Bibliography

Scientific works

Bernstein, Richard K. MD, Dr. Bernstein's Diabetes Solution, 2007
Berry, Ken, MD, Lies my Doctor told Me
Cummins, Ivor and Gerber, Jeffrey, MD, Eat Rich Live Long
Fung, Jason, MD, The Obesity Code
Grundy, Steven R. The Plant Paradox
Kraft, Joseph R. MD, The Diabetes Epidemic & You
Levinovitz, Alan MD, The Gluten Lie
Lustig, Robert MD, Fat Chance
Lustig, Robert MD, The Hacking of the American Mind
Moore, J and Westman, E MD, Cholesterol Clarity
Moore, J and Westman, E MD, Keto Clarity
Mosley, Michael MD, The Fast Life
Noakes, Tim MD, The Lure of Nutrition
Noakes, Tim MD, The Real Meal Revolution
Noakes Foundation, The Banting Pocket Guide
Rheaume-Bleue, K MD, Vitamin K2 & the Calcium Paradox

Wilson, J MD and Lowery, R The Ketogenic Bible

Volek MD and Phinney MD, The Art and Science of Low-Carbohydrate Living

Volek MD and Phinney MD, The Art and Science of Low-Carbohydrate Performance

Culinary works

Artusi, Pellegrino Science in the Kitchen & The Art of Living Well

Healthy Cooking, The Culinary Institute of America

Nutrition, The Culinary Institute of America

Baking for Special Diets, The Culinary Institute of America

Courage, Katherine H., Cultured

Goldwyn, Meathead, Meathead

Morell Sally F., Nourishing Fats

Science Journalism

Taubes, Gary, Good Calories, Bad Calories

Taubes, Gary, Why we Get Fat

Teicholz, Nina, The Big Fat Surprise

Video Resource

Low Carb Down Under (series of conference videos, also contains scientific presentations)

www.ingramcontent.com/pod-product-compliance
Lightning Source LLC
Chambersburg PA
CBHW070340290526
45791CB00003B/1412